Sickle Cell Disease:
Fast Focus Study Guide

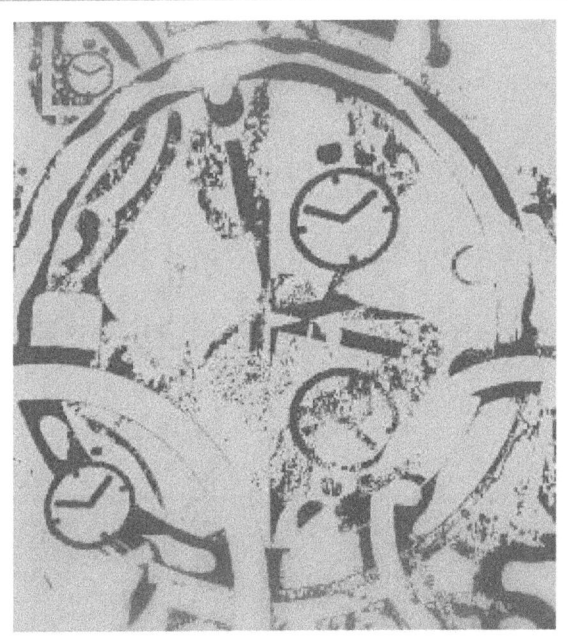

Acknowledgements

I dedicate this book to my beautiful wife and children, who I love more than all the water in all the oceans and all the seas.

CONTENTS

- This book is written for medical professionals who want to learn about Sickle Cell Disease.

- Put this book in your bathroom or on your coffee table.

- This is the perfect graduation gift for the aspiring physician or graduating physician.

- This Fast Focus Study Guide will provide you with a practical review of the key information you need to know.

- Buy this book now if you want this quick and concise information

Patients with sickle cell disease have a hemolytic anemia that is caused by an autosomal recessive defect associated with a single nucleotide substitution in the β globin gene on chromosome 11.

Symptoms of sickle cell often begin at about 4 months of age.

Two hemoglobin S genes are needed to manifest sickle cell disease. The gene is passed down in an autosomal recessive manner. 8-10% of African Americans in the U.S. carry at least one Hgb S gene (sickle cell trait). Approximately 0.15% of African American newborns have sickle cell disease (Hgb SS).

To determine the risk of having a child with sickle cell disease, we have to first determine the risk that each parent will pass along the gene. Two parents that are heterozygous for sickle-cell trait each have a 50% chance of passing on the mutated gene. To calculate the risk of having a child with the disease, we multiply the risk of passing along the gene of each parent. Therefore the risk is 25% (0.5x0.5 = 0.25).

We now have one parent with sickle cell disease (Hgb SS). There is 100% chance that this parent will pass one gene. The other parent has sickle cell trait (Hgb S) and has a 50% chance of passing on a gene. (1x0.5 =0.5). Therefore there is a 50% chance that each child will have sickle cell disease (Hgb SS).

Now let us say we have two parents that are heterozygous (sickle-cell trait) that are having a child. The parents each have a 50% chance of passing on the mutated gene resulting in 25% chance of the disease (0.5x0.5 = 0.25)

The disease severity is variable. Those with sickle cell disease (Hgb SS) have the most symptoms. Those with sickle cell trait (Hgb S) have minimal symptoms if any. Hemoglobin SC disease and Hemoglobin S-beta thal0 disease are more symptomatic than sickle cell trait and less symptomatic than sickle cell disease.

In alpha thalassemia there is decreased Hemoglobin A1 (alpha 2, beta 2) depending on how many of the alpha chain genes (total of 4) are missing or nonfunctional. There is no increase in substitute hemoglobin.

Pain is the most common cause of acute

illness in patients with sickle cell disease.

Additional potential manifestations of sickle cell disease include aplastic crises, splenic sequestration, infection, acute chest syndrome, priapism, stroke, and persistent pain despite proper pain management. Patients can also have priapism, dactylitis, and avascular necrosis of the humeral/femoral head, cholelithiasis, retinopathy, and chronic leg ulcers.

Pain

Acute pain occurs after microvascular occlusion by sickled erythrocytes causes obstruction of blood flow with regional hypoxemia and acidosis. This leads to increased sickling and tissue injury.

Chronic pain results from long term destruction of bones, joints and visceral organs that occurs secondary to recurrent damage from recurrent acute episodes of microvascular occlusion and ischemia.

Patients with acute pain should receive hydration, oxygenation, pain control, and antibiotics if needed. Treatment goals include oxygenation to prevent further sickling. Exchange transfusions can be administered if the simple transfusions do not control symptoms.

Neuropathic pain can occur in patients with sickle cell disease because of nerve injury. Neuropathic pain is characterized by burning, shooting, or tingling sensations.

Non-opioid treatments for mild pain include acetaminophen, nonsteroidal anti-inflammatory drugs (NSAIDs), topical agents, and corticosteroids.

Opioid analgesics can be used for treatment of severe sickle cell associated pain. These medications consist of μ-antagonists (morphine, hydrocodone, oxycodone), mixed agonist /antagonists (butorphanol, dezocine), and antagonists (naloxone, naltrexone, nalmafene).

Hydroxyurea reduces recurrent painful crisis and number of transfusions but is not beneficial during an acute pain episode.

Narcotic addiction is similar in frequency to people with sickle cell disease when compared to people without sickle cell disease.

Anemia

Patients with sickle cell disease have a chronic hemolytic anemia with a baseline compensated anemia at baseline Hb 7-9 g/dl.

Approximately 90% of adults with sickle cell disease will have received at least one RBC transfusion.

The normal life span of RBC is 120 days

sickle cells have average life span of 15 days.

Transfusions are usually not indicated in patients with expected anemia or normal pain.

Patients are generally transfuse for Hb < 5g/dL
if otherwise asymptomatic or <6g/dL with
cardiac decompensation.

Blood transfusions are used for treatment of severe anemia due to acute splenic sequestration, parvovirus B19 infection, or hyper-hemolytic crises. Transfusion is also used in the setting of acute chest syndrome, preoperatively, priapism, and during pregnancy.

Preoperative transfusion support in patients with sickle cell disease is associated with decreased perioperative complications.

Red blood cell transfusions have the potential to help or harm the patient. Potential side effects of transfusion include infection, iron overload, allergic reactions, alloimmunization, and acute or delayed hemolytic transfusion reactions.

The incidence of alloimmunization in patients with sickle cell disease ranges from 18%-76% with ABO and D matching alone.

Approximately 5% of transfused patients with sickle cell disease experience a delayed hemolytic transfusion reaction related to alloimmunization.

The incidence of alloimmunization from red cell transfusions is decreased to 5%-14.5% with limited phenotype matching for C, E, and K antigens and to 7% for extended minor RBC antigen-matching beyond C, E, and K.

More than 90% of Comprehensive Sickle Cell Centers provide red cell transfusions that are matched for C, E, and K to patients with sickle cell disease.

Hyperviscosity and sickle cell complications such as stroke can occur if the patient is transfused much above their baseline hemoglobin. For patients with a baseline hemoglobin above 10 g/ dL should undergo exchange transfusion.

Preoperative transfusion can prevent

intraoperative and postoperative

complications.

Acute Chest Syndrome

Acute chest syndrome is the most common cause of death in patients with sickle cell disease.

National Acute Chest Syndrome Study Group showed that transfusion improves oxygenation.

The treatment of acute chest syndrome includes blood transfusion, respiratory therapy, antibiotics.

Acute chest syndrome treated with transfusion

is associated with shorter hospital stays.

The use of intermittent transfusions for people with acute chest syndrome can result in better outcomes and chronic transfusion treatments in patients with sickle cell can reduce the incidence of acute chest syndrome. Chronic transfusions do not seem to decrease severity of the symptoms.

Exchange transfusions can be used for patients with acute chest syndrome who are not seriously anemic or those with worsening respiratory status or persistent hypoxia even after simple transfusion.

Treatment with Hydroxyurea can be used to prevent recurrent episodes of acute chest syndrome.

Acute chest syndrome occurs because of vaso-occlusive changes in the lungs. Symptoms are characterized by respiratory failure, chest radiograph infiltrate, hypoxia and chest pain. Additional symptoms include cough, dyspnea, or new onset hypoxia.

Acute chest syndrome occurs in 40% of patients with sickle cell disease.

Treatment of acute chest syndrome consists of oxygen, antibiotics, incentive spirometry, simple transfusion, bronchodilators, and pain control without respiratory depression.

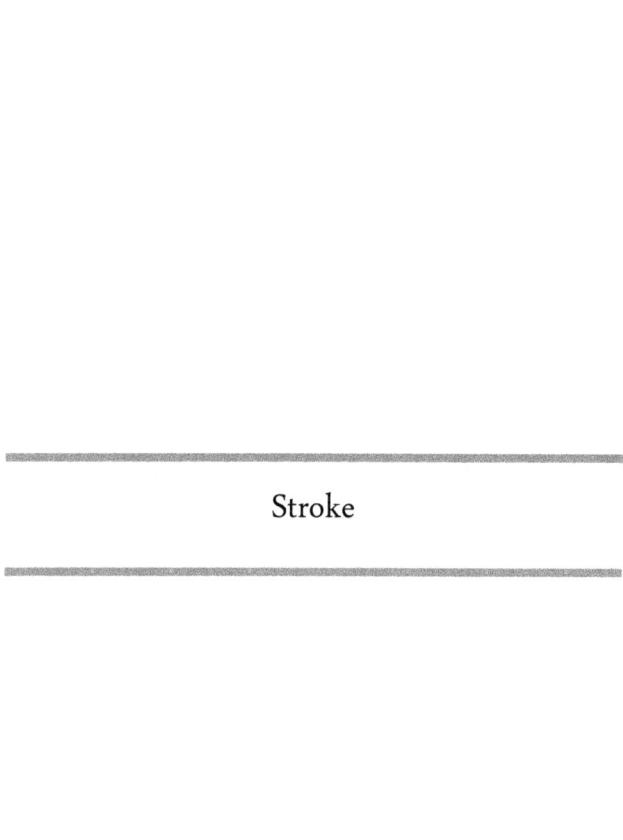

Stroke

Stroke occurs in up to 11% of patients before the age of 20 y/o with peak incidence between 2 and 10 y/o.

Chronic red cell transfusions can reduce the risk of recurrent stroke. Studies show that stroke recurs in about 60% of patients who do not get chronic transfusions and in about 20% of patients who get chronic transfusions to maintain a hemoglobin S percentage of less than 30%.

Acute stroke in patients with sickle cell disease can be treated with red cell transfusion to reduce the percent of hemoglobin S level to below 30%.

Erythrocytapheresis is the most common method of blood transfusion used for initial stroke treatment.

Stroke Prevention Study in Sickle Cell Anemia 2 (STOP 2) demonstrated that chronic transfusion discontinuation results in an increased rate of abnormal transcranial Doppler conversion and stroke.

Exchange transfusion appears to be more effective than simple transfusion for acute treatment and the prevention of secondary stroke.

Stroke symptoms in patients with sickle cell include hemiparesis, palsies, aphasia, seizures or coma.

Acute Splenic Sequestration

Acute splenic sequestration is characterized by a rapid decrease in hemoglobin level with the potential for circulatory shock. Treatment with transfusion needs to be administered carefully because hyperviscosity can occur if red cells in the spleen are remobilized.

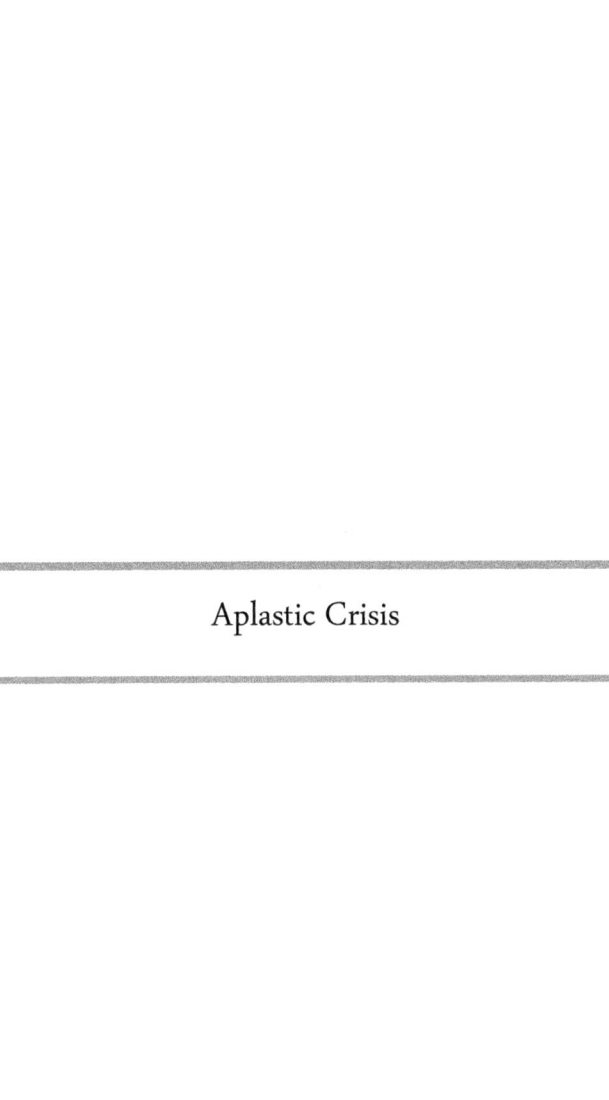

Aplastic Crisis

Aplastic crisis is caused by Parvovirus B19. Patients with sickle cell disease are at risk for this infection which is known to infect young erythrocytes in the bone marrow and decrease production. Symptoms can include fever associated with upper respiratory symptoms.

Priapism

Patients with sickle cell disease are instructed to drink extra fluids, use oral analgesics, and attempt to urinate when priapism develops.

If priapism lasts more than 2 hours the patient is instructed to seek medical attention. Treatment includes intravenous hydration and parenteral pain control. Penile aspiration followed by irrigation of the corpora with a 1:1,000,000 solution of epinephrine in saline is initiated if priapism does not resolve within 1 hour after initiation of medical care.

Red cell exchange transfusions can be performed if the initial therapy is not effective. In cases that still do not resolve a shunt is created between the glans penis and the distal corpora cavernosa allowing blood from the distended corpora cavernosa to drain into the uninvolved corpus spongiosa.

Infection

Young children with sickle cell disease will develop micro infarcts that cause asplenia. Approximately 30% of patients will be asplenic by age 1 and 90% will be asplenic by age 6.

Children with sickle cell disease are at 400 x increased risk for infection with encapsulated organisms such as Streptococcus pneumonia compared to people without sickle cells disease.

Penicillin prophylaxis significantly reduces the incidence of infection with encapsulated organisms.

Protein-conjugated pneumococcal vaccines provide protection against invasive infections are now extensively used.

Salmonella is the most common cause of osteomyelitis in patients with sickle cell disease.

Iron Deficiency

Iron deficiency can occur in patients with sickle cell disease. Intravascular hemolysis can lead to iron loss in sickle cell disease by increased excretion of urinary and biliary iron as hemoglobin, hemosiderin, or heme.

Folic acid deficiency

Folic acid deficiency is prevented with folic acid supplements due to increased folate requirements caused by sickle cell associated hemolysis.

Iron Overload/Secondary Hemochromatosis

A unit of packed red cells contains about 200

mg of iron.

Iron burden can be estimated with ferritin or liver MRI.

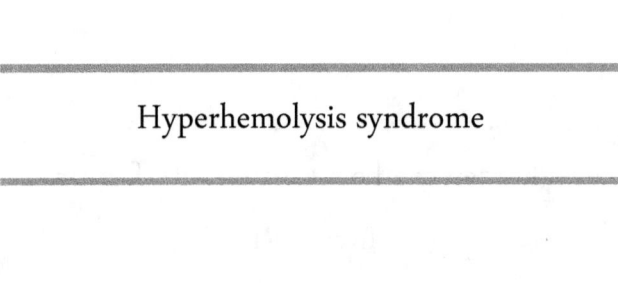

Hyperhemolysis syndrome

Hyperhemolysis syndrome is a characterized in sickle cell disease by a hemoglobin drop lower than the pretransfusion hemoglobin.

Possible mechanisms of hyperhemolysis syndrome include bystander hemolysis, suppression of erythropoiesis, and RBCs being destroyed by activated macrophages.

Treating hyperhemolysis syndrome with transfusion could make things worse. Some patients can be treated with transfusion, corticosteroids and IVIG.

Avascular Necrosis

Avascular necrosis of the femur and humeral head can results from intravascular sickling of red cells in the microcirculation of the bone causing intramedullary sludging causing thrombosis and destruction of the vessel walls. This leads to edema, and worsening ischemia.

MRI is the best imaging modality to diagnose avascular necrosis. Bone scan is not reliable or useful in the diagnosis of avascular necrosis.

Treatment for avascular necrosis includes pain control, heat, and weight bearing restriction. With persistent pain, core decompression of the femoral head can be performed. Hip fusion or reconstruction and total hip replacement can be performed.

Hydroxyurea

Hydroxyurea increases the concentration of fetal hemoglobin and therefore decreases the frequency of sickling. Hydroxyurea also decreases levels of circulating leukocytes, which decreases the adherence of neutrophils to the vascular endothelium.

Hydroxyurea is used in patients with sickle cell disease to treat painful episodes (6 or more per year), acute chest syndrome, severe vaso-occlusive events, symptomatic anemia, chronic pain that cannot be controlled with conservative measure, or a history of stroke or a high risk for stroke.

Hydroxyurea is the most commonly used drug
in use that stimulates HbF production in
patients with sickle cell disease.

Hydroxyurea can decrease the frequency and severity of pain syndromes.

Allogeneic stem cell transplant can be used in the patients with the most severe disease with an event-free survival rate of approximately 84% and a mortality rate of less than 6%.

To be a candidate for an allogeneic stem cell transplant the patient must be younger than 16 years old with HbSS or HbS–β-0 thalassemia with a donor who is a full sibling who is human leukocyte antigen (HLA) compatible (those with sickle trait are acceptable).

Patients who are candidates for stem cell transplant have to have severe disease characterized by stroke, recurrent acute chest syndrome, recurrent priapism, recurrent acute chest syndrome, evidence of cerebral infarction, sickle cell nephropathy, bilateral proliferative retinopathy and major visual impairment in at least one eye, osteonecrosis of multiple joints, or red cell alloimmunization with more than 2 antibodies.

Sickle cell disease occurs due to a structural/qualitative inherited hemoglobin abnormality. Thalassemia is a quantitative inherited hemoglobin abnormality. Sometimes patients can have both abnormalities simultaneously.

Hemoglobin C disease is like hemoglobin S disease (sickle cell) in that both effect the beta globin gene. The gene for hemoglobin C disease is 25% as common as hemoglobin S. Sometimes patients can have both abnormalities, termed hemoglobin SC disease. It is the Second most common hemoglobin variant in Africans and accounts for 1 in 1000 births of African Americans.

The compound heterozygous hemoglobin SC disease is less severe than sickle cell but more severe than sickle cell trait.

Hemoglobin SC has red cells that survive 27 days as compared to the sickle cell hemoglobin cells that survive 17 days.

People with hemoglobin SC disease can have the same problems (splenomegaly, auto splenectomy, veno-occlusive disease, and aseptic necrosis) as people with sickle cell disease, but the severe complications tend to be less frequent.

Beta thalassemia is also characterized by a genetic deficiency in the synthesis of beta-globin chains. In the homozygous state, beta thalassemia (i.e., thalassemia major) causes severe, transfusion-dependent anemia. In the heterozygous state, the beta thalassemia trait (i.e., thalassemia minor) causes mild to moderate microcytic anemia. Sometimes patients can have both a beta thalassemia and a sickle cell gene.

Sickle cell is caused by a mutation of the genes causing an abnormal hemoglobin. Beta thalassemia is characterized by a genetic deficiency in the synthesis of beta-globin chains. The homozygous state, beta thalassemia (ie, thalassemia major) causes severe, transfusion-dependent anemia. The heterozygous state is called beta thalassemia trait (ie, thalassemia minor).

Sickle cell/thalassemia is characterized by a Structural/qualitative problem with hemoglobin because of a mutant DNA that creates a beta chain that does not work well and beta thalassemia has a quantitative problem because it does not making enough hemoglobin because one or more of the beta chains are reduced or absent.

Beta thalassemia is one-tenth as common as sickle cell anemia.

Sickle cell-beta thalassemia is divided into sickle cell-beta0 (thalassemia major) thalassemia and sickle cell-beta+ (thalassemia minor), based upon the complete absence beta globin or the presence of reduced amounts of beta globin.

Patients with sickle cell-beta0 thalassemia have no HbA production and have a clinical course as severe as homozygous sickle cell disease.

Patients with sickle cell-beta+ thalassemia are have a low HbA production. These people generally have a less severe disease than either sickle cell anemia or sickle cell-beta0 thalassemia.

Alpha thalassemia results from a defect in the production of alpha globin chains causing a relative excess of beta globin chains. Clinical manifestations are generally less severe in sickle cell-alpha thalassemia compared with sickle cell-beta thalassemia.

Sickle cell-alpha thalassemia is associated with a milder anemia with fewer reticulocytes and sickled cells.

Patients with sickle cell alpha thalassemia have hemoglobin A2 levels that are increased according to the number of alpha globin gene deletions. Hemoglobin F levels are not consistently affected.

The hemoglobin electrophoresis in patients with SC disease will show equal amounts of HbS and HbC (or slightly more HbS than HbC), with no HbA present and rarely will the fetal hemoglobin be greater than 50%.

These are the 3 normal types of hemoglobin

Hemoglobin A- alpha (2), beta (2)

Hemoglobin A2- alpha (2), delta (2)

Hemoglobin F- alpha (2), gamma (2)

The following page outlines the expected

hemoglobin ratios in various diseases.

Sickle cell trait will have a HbS
concentrations of 35 to 45% of total
Hemoglobin.

Alpha thalassemia with Sickle cell trait will have a HbS concentrations of <33% of total Hemoglobin.

S-Beta-thalassemia or Sickle cell disease with transfusion will have a HbS concentrations of >50% of total Hemoglobin.

Hemoglobin A2 will be decreased in iron deficiency, alpha-thalassemia.

Hemoglobin A2 will be elevated in megaloblastic anemia, hyperthyroidism, and beta-thalassemia.

Hemoglobin F will be increased in sickle cell anemia and Beta thalassemia major.

Carefully review the following hemoglobin

electrophoresis

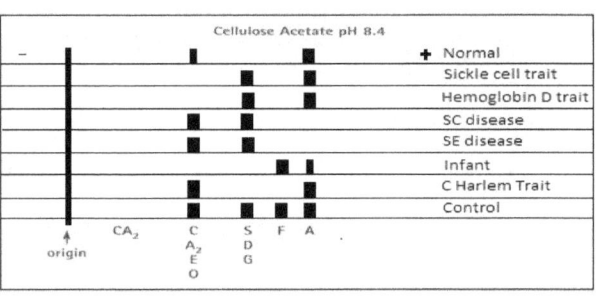

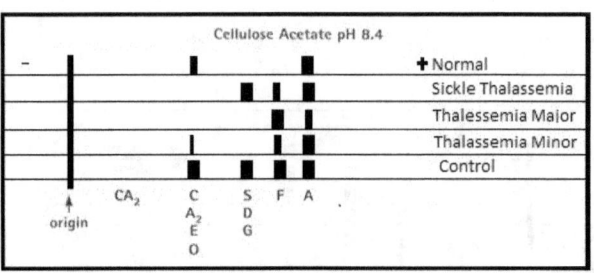

This concludes Sickle Cell Disease: Fast Focus Study Guide

Search Amazon Kindle books to find other study guides written by

JT Thomas, MD

Internal Medicine Study Guide

Hematology Study Guide

Medical Oncology Study Guide

Multiple Myeloma Study Guide

Differential Diagnosis Study Guide